How To Be *LESS* Fat (and Live Better, Longer)

by James Dertian

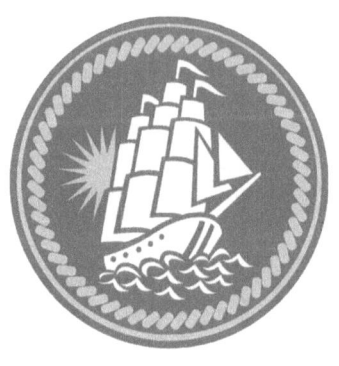

Galleon Publishing
Atlanta, GA

GALLEON SELF-DEVELOPMENT

TABLE OF CONTENTS

Introduction & Disclaimer

I am 32 years old, 6 feet tall and weigh 265 pounds. By almost every measure, my body is beyond what is considered a normal or healthy weight for my height.

Not beating around the bush here... I'm obese!

My Body Mass Index (BMI) is well over 30 right now. That's not a good number.

It's football season and earlier today I ate three slices of pizza. Plus, I drank two regular beers. Not light beers mind you; they were full-calorie regular beers that were absolutely delicious. And there were meat-based toppings on the pizza, a small fistful of pork and beef bits. Might have even had "extra cheese" on there too, I'm not sure.

My team lost, but I enjoyed (and indulged) myself fully.

Naturally, you must be wondering what the hell business a fat guy like me has writing a book about weight loss. I mean c'mon, it's more than a fair question.

Well, I'll tell you. As a matter of fact, I'm more than a little proud of myself. Over the last 2 years I've lost nearly 100 pounds with a surprisingly limited amount of exercise and dieting. The quality of my life has improved tremendously, and while I'm still quite overweight, I actually feel FANTASTIC.

This book is not peddling some moronic miracle cure. I don't want you to start sprinkling magic powder on the food you eat and I'm not going to encourage you to start drinking wheatgrass juice and doing intense yoga six times a week. This is a book about what it takes to lose weight, in practical terms.

I'm writing this for people who are still living the life I was trapped in just a couple of short years ago. People who wake up and feel bad from the very moment they step out of bed. Maybe it's not an overt misery, but being massively overweight drags you down in every single facet of your life.

As a disclaimer, I guess I should make a few things clear. **First off, you must consult your doctor before embarking on any weight loss plan or program.** This book is not really advocating a specific or directed weight loss program, per se, but if you're going to try to drop some weight – talking to your doctor is always the place you're supposed to start. I am definitely not a doctor.

Also, the things I will be talking about in this book apply if you're 40 pounds overweight or if you're 400 pounds overweight. But as you can probably guess, I'm not writing for the somewhat slender woman who wants to drop 5 pounds by next month so she can wear her favorite dress to the company Christmas party. If that's you, go hit up any magazine rack.

But First, My Confession…

James Dertian is a pen name that I have chosen to use while writing this short e-book. The reason I have elected to use a name based on my real name and not my actual name is sort of complicated. But let me try to explain.

In this book I wanted to have the freedom to be pretty frank about my own struggles with weight and my personal shortcomings. I have written under a pen name because, probably much like yourself, I have a full time day job and want to keep it.

I am not writing this book to launch a fitness revolution or to make millions. It's likely you purchased this title on Amazon or another online book retailer for no more than a dollar or two, which is enough to cover the costs of the publisher, put a few cents in the retailer's pocket and filter down a little change my way.

I am not going to try to sell you a weight loss system. I am not going to write any other books or teach any classes or go on television. This book is not a first step to some integrated fitness empire of DVDs and radio interviews and video game tie-ins. All of that stuff is crap, designed not to help you lose weight, but to help you spend money.

Despite what you might assume, I don't enjoy talking about my weight loss. Partly, because I'm not really thin, I've just lost a lot of weight. I also feel quite a bit of shame about how much of my life was pissed away by being extremely obese.

My whole reason for writing this is to reach out to other people who are still in that category. It's a rapidly growing segment of the population, sadly. Being morbidly obese is locked being locked in a prison that you carry around on your back. If I can help even one person to get motivated to break out of that prison, then this little book will have been a huge success.

How Did I Get Here?

I obviously know that eating fewer calories means losing more weight. It's common sense and it's what I always tell people when they pitch me some goofy diet involving only meat, or eating between certain hours of the day or whatever. But knowing and using that information are two different things, and for whatever crazy, self-destructive reason... I just never controlled myself.

People use food to regulate their emotions. For a long time, I think I was eating as a way to fill an empty hole inside. Then there's social motivation. When you surround yourself with fat, unhealthy people it becomes socially acceptable for you to engage in these behaviors. I did a lot of that, seeking out people and sharing the misery.

More than 10 years ago, when I graduated from high school, I weighed 208 pounds. The summer before I graduated, I had gotten down to about 185-190 pounds and was wearing a size medium t-shirt. After graduation, I moved out on my own and the eating just got WAAAY out of control.

I remember that I once ate two large pizzas... in the same evening. It was just out of control binge eating.

I would order from Taco Bell up to 6 times a week! I'd make DAILY trips to the grocery store to get provisions... fish sticks, candy bars, frozen pizzas, cookies, pies, ice cream.

If I was low on money, I'd basically keep up my behavior, but lower my standards. Instead of ordering delivery or going to the "nice" supermarket and getting deli meats and premium ice cream, I would head over to Food Lion or another discount grocery store. I'd buy the cheapest frozen pizza and a tube of raw cookie dough. I sought out just enough food to totally fill me up and make me feel sick enough to fall asleep.

Seriously, I was pretty screwed up in those early days. It was like attempted suicide by food. Except, it didn't feel that way at the time. It was more like if someone had offered me a job eating food, and it was just what I had to do... get a ton of food and eat it. Fall asleep, wake up, and get a ton of food again.

As I said, when I graduated high school, I was at 208 pounds. By the end of the summer, I was up to around 225 and pushing 250 by the end of that year.

By then I was living on the other side of the country from where I'd grown up, I only had work friends, lived in a very tiny apartment, and food became my after work release.

The summer before food was my daily job. Now it was a drug. I'd get off work and go shoot-up a gigantic bowl of spaghetti. And on Friday evening? Well, holy shit... it was ON! Some people couldn't wait for the weekend so they could go party and get drunk. I couldn't wait for the weekend so I could go home, change into my elastic waist pants, and sit in front of the computer/television while consuming TREMENDOUS amounts of food.

By the time I decided to leave my job and the state of California, and return home to go back to college, I was tipping the scales at 290 pounds.

I got home in September of 2001, just before the terrorist attacks. By Christmas I had hit 300.

And then, a pause.

I didn't gain any weight for about a year. Or rather, it took a whole year to go from 300 to 305 pounds.

It was a slow but steady climb from December 2002 to December 2004... at which point I'd reached 330 pounds. I would lose 10 or 15 pounds over a few months, then go and gain 20.

In 2005, I actually controlled myself a little and got back down to 315. I thought maybe I was getting myself together. But it wasn't to last.

After college, I went to work, met someone, and by the time of my wedding in 2009 I weighed 360 pounds.

I was eating probably 4,000 or more calories a day and barely exercising at all to make up for it. On my way to 400 pounds and an early grave, I finally decided that enough HAD to be enough.

If You Think I'm Fat Now...

So there I was, 360 pounds of goo. My 20s should have been some of the best years of my life, but my food addiction and self-destructive behavior robbed me of most of that decade.

I wore 3XLT shirts, not so much because I was "tall" and needed the T, but because I really needed to be wearing 4XL shirts and getting the "tall" version of the 3XL was allowing me to delude myself just a little bit.

When you're as monumentally fat as I was, you'll take every drop of false encouragement that you can get.

The economic destruction my morbid obesity wreaked on my life was absolutely immeasurable. People complain that it "costs more" to eat healthy, but let me tell you that is total, unmitigated bullshit.

It costs a ton of money to be super- fat, like I was.

No, I don't mean that food is expensive... although it definitely can be. And I'm not just talking about doctor bills or having to buy 2 seats on an airplane in order to fly somewhere, although that does play into the equation.

The real economic cost of being huge is in lost income. I guess that somehow I never realized it while I was gaining all that weight, but people treat the morbidly obese like they're unreliable and untrustworthy.

In some ways, I really can understand the thought process. Having made the journey more than half-way down Fat Mountain, I now find myself looking at the folks who are pushing 400 pounds and wondering about their character. What's wrong with them? What was wrong with me? It's sad, but true.

From an employer's perspective, if I had a choice between hiring me now and hiring me from 2 years ago, there would be no comparison. At my extreme weight, I often found it difficult to focus. I was hugely uncomfortable in social situations. I just wasn't a good employee.

The amount of work I got done in any given day back when I weighed 350+ pounds was probably half of what I can now complete as I'm approaching 250 pounds. My energy was just totally drained by carrying around the giant lump of butter that was my body.

I lost out on job opportunities, I lost out on promotions. I wasted years of my life, what should have been some of the most productive years of my life, going nowhere because of how enormously fat I used to be. That's time and potential that I will never recover.

Throw Away Your Goals!

For years when I weighed over 350 pounds I had it stuck in my mind that I needed to get back down to 190 pounds in order to be happy.

That was how much I weighed towards the end of high school.

Truthfully, I looked pretty good at that weight. Girls were interested in me, to some degree. No one treated me as being particularly overweight. I was just a normal person.

If it wasn't possible to recapture that feeling, then what was the point of losing weight? What good would it do?

The trip back to 190 pounds from over 350 was just too much to wrap my mind around. Any way I sliced it, it would take years to come even close. The whole situation felt totally hopeless, and so I'd head to the freezer for an ice cream sandwich.

Being so far away from my goal weight would cause me to fixate only on the more radical dieting options. After watching an excellent documentary on Netflix about a guy who went on a juice fast, I decided that I'd finally found the answer!

Unfortunately, I lacked the willpower to complete the 10 day fast I started out with and that failure just lead me to eat more and more. Feeling sorry for myself, I'd dive into gigantic portions of Mexican food with total disregard. It was almost like I was punishing myself for the failure of my juice fast. Crazy thinking.

What I eventually learned is that if you are extremely overweight, like me, your goal can't be to lose 100 pounds. You shouldn't try to radically change your life overnight and go from a diet of all McDonald's to one of only salads and fresh fruit. It's a ridiculous proposition and it only sets you up for more failure, more depression and more eating.

I know. I spent a decade chowing down and sitting around while my life went nowhere. My extreme weight cost me job opportunities, it cost me relationships. There were huge parts of my youth that I experienced only through a foggy window.

It's not possible to really enjoy college when you're north of 300 pounds.

It's not possible to have a great first day at work when your desk chair cuts into your big fat sides and you're totally winded after carrying some things up to your office.

If you live in a warm climate, like I did, then you sweat all day long and your whole life is just miserable.

Dotted throughout that period in my life were little initiatives. I'd go on a juice fast or the Atkins Diet. I'd try Nutrisystem and get stuck paying for a bunch of horrible freeze dried food, half of which went into the trash can. It was like being a crazy person who would have an occasional moment of lucidity.

One day, I would wake up and realize how dire my situation was and get to work trying to fix it. I'd join a gym or start lifting weights in my basement. A week or two later, I'd descend back into my food fog, depressed by my slow progress. I might lose 5 pounds in a week and then gain 10 in the month that followed.

The biggest thing standing in my way of real, lasting weight loss was this huge goal. It seemed like setting more realistic goals was the answer to my prayers.

People told me that if I just targeted a smaller goal, I could stay motivated until I achieved it.

Listen, maybe goal setting works for some people. Judging from our society's growing waistlines, however, I think it's safe to say that goal-centric weight loss just isn't cutting it. Whether you have a huge long-term weight loss goal or some shorter term targets, most people who try to work towards weight loss goals *fail miserably*.

It was only when I finally dumped all my goals that I began to achieve any kind of lasting progress.

Free yourself from these silly prisons. Throw your goals into the garbage!

Don't try to lose 100 pounds by next year. Don't try to drop 20 pounds in time for summer. Just stop. Wipe your mind clear of this nonsense.

Forgive yourself for failing. Let yourself off the hook.

And then we can get to work.

FAT FACT

According to a recent report on overweight and obesity published by the office of the U.S. Surgeon General, women gaining more than 20 pounds between age 18 and midlife double their risk of postmenopausal breast cancer compared with women whose weight remains stable.

(Source: Obesity in America)

Privacy Worked For Me...

The conventional wisdom is that your new diet or exercise program will have a better chance of success if you announce to all of your family and friends that you're undertaking it.

Articles and weight loss gurus talk about posting your workout routines and weight loss results on Facebook and Twitter. I guess the thinking is that telling your coworkers about your new healthy eating and active lifestyle will sort of shame you into staying on the diet.

The experts call it making yourself accountable, and maybe it does work for some people. I was not in that category. Whenever I told people I was going on a diet the responses I would get would range from encouragement to indifferent shrugs.

As each dieting push failed and a new one began, I got more and more indifferent shrugs. People were expecting me to fail and the whole dynamic served as a de-motivator for me.

Here's the truth. I lost all of my weight by keeping my damn mouth shut -- and I don't just mean eating less!

Talking about weight loss doesn't lead to weight loss; all that talk just causes you to fixate on how difficult the change you're trying to make is. As well intentioned as my wife was, whenever I told her I was going on a diet she would begin to immediately nag and annoy me about everything I ate that wasn't a celery stick. It was actually making me resent her, resent the diet and causing significant and needless stress on our relationship. I would start binge eating in private, a horrible habit.

Maybe being very public about a diet works for some people, but it sure wasn't working for me!

I've told my wife and my friends before that I was going to try exercising. I've started taking salads and blended vegetable juices to work for lunch. People knew I was struggling to lose weight and it just made my eventual failures all the more painful. Once everyone knew I was on a diet, I almost couldn't wait to sabotage myself to just get the whole thing over with and put it all in the past.

If you want to lose weight, I believe that you need to internalize the plan and internalize the pain. It's not about your friends and family, they can't lose the weight for you.

This is all about you.

FAT FACT

Between 1980 and 2000, obesity rates doubled among adults. About 60 million adults, or 30% of the adult population, are now obese.

Similarly since 1980, overweight rates have doubled among children and tripled among adolescents – increasing the number of years they are exposed to the health risks of obesity.

(Source: Centers for Disease Control)

Dieting is Dumb...

I consumed well over 4,000 calories on a daily basis just to maintain my weight. Cutting back my calorie intake by even 10% would cause me to start losing about a pound a week without any other effort. But when I tried this approach, I found that counting the calories make me feel like I was rationing.

When people start off dieting with a goal, the goal is generally to be a thin and happy person.

One of the things that I really want to share with you is that a diet can still be successful, even if you fall very short of that "ultimate happiness" goal. But the reality is that you should never diet and you should not set these types of unreachable goals.

If you want to change your life, you need to change your lifestyle.

Here's What I Did...

Scientists and disaster movies have long dwelled on the possibility that a rogue asteroid in outer space might be discovered on a collision course with the planet Earth.

In the disaster movies, NASA seems to focus on blowing up the space rock at the last minute with nuclear bombs that are launched inside rockets or that are delivered by a crew of roughneck astronauts who save humanity in fantastic fashion.

The Hollywood approach to asteroid destruction is similar to how most people think of dieting.

The day is saved by a small amount of expensive, focused effort directed at the oncoming rock. It is blown to smithereens and all of our problems are solved!

Roll credits.

The reality, and what actually could save us from an asteroid, is something very different than these high octane big screen stunts.

Every day, scientists are combing the skies and calculating the trajectories of new objects that they discover. It seems inevitable that at some point they'll find a big rock that is headed our way. When that does happen, NASA won't be calling Bruce Willis or Clint Eastwood to come save the day.

The best way to protect Earth is to address the problem as early as possible, reaching the asteroid years before it poses a direct danger to the planet. Then, you simply attach a small rocket to the big rock and alter the asteroid's trajectory a little bit. Over the span of several years, that small course correction will grow and grow exponentially, sending the object harmlessly hurtling past our pale blue dot. It doesn't make for a particularly exciting movie, but it's a vastly cheaper and safer way to handle such a threat.

I applied the same thinking to weight loss. Throwing out those big, bold goals I mentioned earlier, instead I favored small and sensible changes in my everyday patterns of behavior. I sought out things that would slowly, steadily alter my course over time.

What you need to do initially is to break the absolute worst of your bad behaviors. For me, that was binge eating in private. After work I would often hit a fast food restaurant drive-through window and consume perhaps 500-600 calories during the 10 minute ride home. Then I'd clean myself up and walk in the door like nothing had happened.

An hour later, my wife and I would both eat normal looking dinners and I would make no mention of my Big Mac pre-dinner snack.

You might not have the serious binge eating problem that I had, but I bet you have some horrible habits of your own.

MAKING COURSE CORRECTIONS

The very first change I made was to stop all of my eating at or around midnight. Because of an unusual work schedule, I often went to bed around 3am and got up at about 9am. I knew that I did approximately 20% of my eating during those last three-hours of my day, usually while I sat around and watched television or screwed around on the computer. Those three hours were certainly the least productive and most destructive of my entire day.

I didn't adjust anything else about my diet at first, except for the period between midnight and 3am.

This is a variation on a common piece of weight loss advice that says you shouldn't eat any food for a certain number of hours before you go to sleep.

My results were fantastic. Instead of going to sleep at 3am and getting 6 hours of decent sleep, I would suddenly be in the mood to hit the sack by 1am. I was enjoying a full eight hours of high quality sleep and waking up with much more energy.

The change happened within just a few days, this isn't something that took weeks or months to start paying me dividends.

The problem with the standard advice about not eating X-number of hours before bed is that, as you go to sleep earlier, you have to stop eating even earlier. And since you can't just sleep all day long, it's a bit harder to manage. It feels restricting.

I found that the midnight rule made a huge difference in my life. It also helped that I would allow myself to bend the rule once or twice a month if I was legitimately hungry. It was better that the rule be allowed to bend than for it to break apart completely.

Most of my eating between midnight and 3am was out of boredom, not real hunger. Once I had recognized that in myself, I saw the opportunity to change something.

The final result was that I would eat more than I used to before midnight, but less food overall for the entire day. In addition to the extra sleep and energy, I estimated that had probably cut my daily caloric intake by 5-10%. It made a significant difference.

I began to lose a few pounds with what felt like minimal effort. I was less bloated, less tired and much less miserable. That's the point where I decided to make another change, this time coming in the form of physical activity. My new energy needed an outlet, so

I began planning day trips for myself and my wife on Saturdays. In the past we might have sat around all day watching TV or gone out to the movies and a restaurant, but now I was determined to start moving a little bit.

We visited a few national parks and monuments that were within a couple hours of our home. One day we went fishing, which I admit is not a very physically taxing exercise, but when you compare it to sitting in a lump on the couch it made a night and day difference.

FAT FACT

Obesity threatens to overwhelm our health care system.

• 80% of Type II diabetes is related to obesity
• 70% of cardiovascular disease related to obesity
• 30% of gall bladder surgery related to obesity

National costs attributed to illnesses with ties to overweight and obesity accounted for 9.1 percent of total U.S. medical expenditures in 1998 and may have reached as high as $78.5 billion. That number has been steadily climbing over the past decade and a half.

(Source: The Get Fit America Foundation)

Weight Loss is a Momentum Game

Weight loss and politics are very similar. There are a whole lot of lies involved, and a bunch of wasted money.

The most important factor in elections, it has been often said, is momentum. The candidate with momentum going into Election Day almost always wins.

It's really amazing how much momentum plays into our weight. Positive momentum often leads you to do better and better, but let negative momentum take over and it can spiral into a deadly crash on chocolate fudge mountain faster than I could swallow a pair of McDonald's double cheeseburgers.

When I got started with my efforts to change my eating habits, I began by cutting back on calories in a casual way for well over three months before the changes were even noticed by any friends or family members.

It was a ton of effort at first, but over time things became easier and easier. Having the wind in your sails makes you stand up just a bit taller and smile just a bit brighter.

My wife never really thought I was on a diet because I was still eating cake and pizza and all this stuff just like she would normally see me eat. But eventually she did notice I was losing weight, and the little positive comments from everyone around me added fuel to my slow burning fire.

Instead of being on a secret binge, I was on a secret diet.

At work, I'd still go to the company picnic BBQ. I'd still go out to drinks with friends. Hell, I remember a couple of times when I went out with friends and I had a big steak and a scotch without any real reservation. If the situation called for it, I would eat or drink whatever was required.

But the pounds kept falling off, bit by bit, because I was being diligent about cutting out the food that other people didn't see. The biggest reductions I made were to my "alone eating" -- the excessive late night snacking at first. And the Big Macs before dinner had to go as well. I just made a game of it, slashing back this low value, high calorie fast food I was eating.

The more weight I would drop, the better I would feel about myself and the more positive feedback I would get from the world.

I say feedback from the world, because the experience is not just about getting encouragement from friends and family. A huge part of the feedback you experience is silent. You go to the movies and the seat is more comfortable. You have to fly somewhere and suddenly the embarrassing question of buying 2 seats is no longer a concern. You go outside on a hot day and it takes an extra couple minutes before you begin to sweat. It's all of these little things -- that occur all day long -- that make you feel better about your body and yourself.

At my new not-so-thin weight of 265 pounds, I can go to concerts and sold-out movies without the fear of having to sit directly next to someone in a tight seat. When I was north of 350 pounds, every single event I attended was a nightmare.

Once you're moving in the right direction and making noticeable progress with your weight loss efforts, the momentum becomes intoxicating.

High-Value Foods

In this section, I'm going to talk about eating smart, high-value foods in order to help you lose weight.

In a normal "diet" book, that would mean explaining the value of nuts and whole grain and how you can drink lots of water to feel full. But that's not exactly what I mean by high-value foods.

You see, when I was extremely fat, I would eat huge amounts of food that I loved and huge amounts of food that just happened to be in front of me.

I'd order some Italian food for delivery from my favorite place, and then to kill time while I was waiting for the 40 minute delivery I would go make myself a sandwich or eat an ice cream cone or something. And then when I was done with my Italian food, I'd go have another ice cream cone for dessert. The chicken parmesan was bad, but the food I was eating around it was so much worse for me.

Why was I eating like this? It was boredom, probably. I sought out food to feel happy; shoveling whatever was around into my mouth into order to achieve that momentary high.

My new lifestyle has caused me to take a serious inventory of how I eat, and now I pick and choose what is really important to me. It's like the question of what would you take from your house if it was on fire and you only had a moment to grab some personal belongings.

I kept Thanksgiving dinner in full force, no Tofurky for me.

I kept pizza and beer on football afternoons with friends.

Instead, I cut those horrible Big Macs after work. I cut out the late night boredom eating. There were thousands of calories in my diet every week that were based around boredom and bad scheduling, not hunger.

REAL HUNGER

"Fake it till you make it" is something they often say in the entertainment industry. It works for weight loss as well. I acted more and more like a normal person until suddenly, the weight was falling off and the act became reality.

Instead of trying to eat a bunch of salad all week long, I just chose to eat like a normal person when I was around my friends and family. Having three slices of pizza instead of four doesn't make a difference in your weight... if you do it one time. But if you make it the rule, after a year of skipping the extra piece of pizza, you WILL have something to show for it.

In the old days, I never stopped eating long enough to feel truly hungry. I'm here to tell you that hunger isn't a bad thing, necessarily.

I find it empowering now, to get up and feeling legitimately hungry before I eat anything is a joy. It's not painful. I feel lighter on my feet, my bones and muscles feel better. There is nothing to fear from a little dose of hunger now and then.

HIGH-VALUE FOODS?

So, what are these high-value foods? Honestly, that's something you will have to decide for yourself. They are different for everyone.

People drive themselves crazy on diets, fixating on trying to get through Thanksgiving dinner or a 4th of July BBQ without overeating. But those are one-time events. The calories you should be attacking are the everyday garbage.

The easiest way to identify your high-value foods is to do this little exercise: If I told you that you would have to go on a strict diet starting tomorrow, what comes to mind as being the most painful part of that diet? What are you going to miss the most?

For me, it was big family meals once or twice a week. It was food while watching sports. It was holidays. In my mind, those were going to be the biggest bummers of a new, restricting diet. So, with those high-value foods in mind, I set about cutting only from the low-value column.

What I came up with was fast food, impulse buying candy at the gas station and boredom eating late at night. That food wasn't really that valuable to me. I was eating it out of compulsion and habit, but it was doing the most damage.

FAT FACT

New research suggests that a few extra pounds or a slightly larger waistline affects an executive's perceived leadership ability as well as stamina on the job.

Executives with larger waistlines and higher body-mass-index readings tend to be perceived as less effective in the workplace, both in performance and interpersonal relationships, according to data compiled by the Center for Creative Leadership. BMI, a common measure of body fat, is based on height and weight.

A heavy executive is judged to be less capable because of assumptions about how weight affects health and stamina, says Barry Posner, a leadership professor at Santa Clara University's Leavey School of Business. He says he can't name a single overweight Fortune 500 CEO. "We have stereotypes about fat," he adds, "so when we see a senior executive who's overweight, our initial reaction isn't positive."

(Source: The Wall Street Journal)

Let's Do Some Calorie Math

First off, it's important that we understand what a calorie actually is.

Calories are a unit of energy that was first identified in the 1800s. Technically, a calorie is the amount of heat needed to raise the temperature of 1 gram of water by 1 degree Celsius. But that's the science book definition. In the everyday world, a calorie is the potential energy in food and the amount of energy the body uses. It is the currency of your physical life and strength.

You consume calories and then you burn them for fuel.

Calories are comprised of three types of nutrients, which are carbohydrates, fats and proteins. Sounds familiar, right?

Water, vitamins and minerals are all free of calories.

When we take in food, the energy we don't need to utilize immediately is stored as body fat, regardless of the nutrient it comes from. That means excess carbohydrates are no more fattening than additional calories from any source, including fats and proteins.

Which weighs more, a pound of iron or a pound of feathers?

It works the same with calories... eating 1,000 calories of ice cream and eating 1,000 calories of tofu are both still adding 1,000 calories to your diet.

CALORIES PER POUND

The other big piece of the equation is that there are approximately 3,500 calories in every pound of body fat. In simple terms, that means if you are 100 pounds overweight you've built up a 350,000 calorie reserve in your body. Instead of money in the bank, think of that stash of calories as a huge debt that you owe. You've charged up 350,000 calories on the credit card of your of body and now you need to begin paying that off.

To the extent that I've done any counting in my weight loss push over the last two years, it's been all about calories. Because calories are the only thing that matter.

It's insane, but there is a billion dollar industry of weight loss schemes in this country that spend all of their time trying to trick and confuse us all. They suggest that weight loss is a very difficult to understand dark art. Weight Watchers, Jenny Craig and Nutrisystem all want you to believe that this is far more complicated than it really is.

TRUST ME: You don't need to pay them for the answer!

FAT FACT

Registered dietitian Jill Weisenberger tells her clients that calories are money. "You have a certain amount in your budget, and if you spend too much, you go into debt. If you take more than your calorie allowance, you get fat."

If you want extra money for something special, you might try to earn more or save.

"Think of calories the same way: If you want some extra for a special dessert or other treat, earn them by doing extra exercise, or save them from another time," Weisenberger said. "A 500-calorie slice of cheesecake will take an hour or more of really hard exercise. Or you could skip that second piece of buttered toast at breakfast, cut your juice in half and trade in your large sandwich for a smaller one. Or you could combine dietary and exercise changes."

(Source: The Los Angeles Times)

Activity is Important (Obviously)

It's embarrassing, but I've probably started a half-dozen weight loss programs by rushing out and joining a gym, only to have the membership fee taken from my account each month without me ever setting foot in the building. I might go for a week or two at the start, but once I stopped going, it was nearly impossible to get back into the habit. And the shame I felt every time the fee was debited from my bank account only caused me to want to go eat a sandwich.

Here's a secret: the gyms love this! Most gyms in this country would be forced out of business if they made all of their money from people who actually went there and worked out. A huge portion of their income comes from these one and two year contracts that are started by well-meaning people.

Every day you don't go to the gym is a day that you're not wearing out their equipment and taking up space. The most profitable gym members, by far, are the ones who sign a long contract and then never use the facility after the first couple of sessions.

As I described earlier, once I had begun to lose weight by cutting out some of the calories in my diet that weren't really important to me, I noticed a surge of energy. I think using that surge of energy to begin exercise is a great "phase 2" of your weight loss plan of attack, which is slowly ramping up your level of overall physical activity.

So don't go out and join some gym. Instead, when that energy level starts to perk up after you lose a few pounds, jump on it and harness it to help you accelerate your progress.

If you are extremely overweight, then odds are good that you're at least a part-time couch potato. I was a master spud, myself!

I started scheduling activities for myself and my wife on the weekend, but you might find a morning walk is more your speed. Whatever works for you, do more and more of it.

Instead of joining a gym or buying a bunch of expensive exercise equipment, I spent about $20 on a nice 25 pound dumbbell at Wal-Mart. It was all one piece, small and easy to store in my home office's closet. Around midnight, when I stopped eating for the day, I would grab the dumbbell and do about 3 minutes of curls and other exercises. Think about that amount of time – just three minutes! That's 180 seconds. It's nothing in the big scheme of your day, but doing those minutes with the weights would tire me out a little bit and, after a week or two, it became incredibly easy. I could feel myself growing stronger and it caused me to expand my time with the weights to five minutes.

After about six months, I purchased a 35 pound dumbbell to partner up with my original 25 pound weight. Every night I use these two weights for between three and eight minutes. If I miss a day for some reason, I'll do 2 sessions the next day to make up for it.

That's it for me, though. I own no other exercise equipment and I have not joined a gym.

My "workout routine" is nothing more than five minutes of weights at night, a long walk once or twice a week, and getting out and staying on my feet doing fun activities during the weekend.

A couple of months ago I had a nice backyard bar-b-que with a few friends and family coming over to my house. I ate at least two hot dogs and a hamburger, but I probably didn't gain much weight that day. I had to haul the grill out of the garage, clean it, and then spent well over an hour standing over the fire cooking the food while interacting with people. All that effort was burning calories.

The old me would probably have suggested we all get together and go to a bar-b-que restaurant to pig out. Or worse, I probably wouldn't have organized any activity and would instead have spent that Saturday sitting in front of the TV or the computer and having pizza delivered.

Moving around doesn't have to be painful, it can actually be quite a lot of fun.

Some small changes in how you live can yield huge results over time.

Being Less Fat is Awesome

I am not thin, nor am I even at a healthy weight for my height. But I am well on my way, and even if I didn't lose another pound after today, as long as I don't gain it all back, I'll have won.

I've learned how important it is to free yourself from the prison of expectations. Diets don't work; changing your lifestyle is the only thing that can lead to lasting happiness. Cutting out those low-value foods we talked about and understanding the nature of calories and the scams perpetrated by the weight loss industry, so you don't fall into their traps.

Keep repeating it in your head: *Eat less, move more! Fake it till you make it!*

Being LESS FAT is like getting your life back, with training wheels. Every five or ten pounds lost brings with it a new treat. I have more stamina in the bedroom. I notice the seatbelt in my car fits better; my office chair is no longer snug around my waist. People look at me so much differently, it just blows me away.

If you're like I was, if you're exhausted from being fat… know that there is hope. There is joy in ANY weight loss, even if you don't wind up looking like a super model.

This is literally a matter of life and death. They don't call it being "morbidly" obese because you live a long time. At 370 pounds, I probably wouldn't have seen my 50th birthday. Or if I did make it, I might well have had to undergo heart surgery or some other invasive and horrendous surgical procedure.

Now that I am less fat, I have bought myself more time. I am living better and loving my life. I plan to continue my journey by starting a family and trying to keep the weight loss momentum going in my favor. It's exciting, and much easier than I ever expected.

I hope you make the choice to join me.

Resources to Get Started

Calorie King Calculator:
http://www.calorieking.com/interactive-tools/weight-maintenance-calories-calculator/

This awesome free calculator lets you enter your gender, height and weight to get a relatively accurate estimate of how many calories you're currently burning in a single day. Use this number as a baseline guide when estimating how many calories you've cut from your diet.

Fast Food That Won't Kill You:
http://www.fitnessmagazine.com/recipes/healthy-eating/on-the-go/healthy-fast-foods/

This article in *Fitness* magazine outlines 24 not terrible fast food options from KFC, McDonald's, Taco Bell, Wendy's and Pizza Hut. Having a few semi-healthy options in mind can be a huge help if you find yourself in a social situation where fast food is the only option. For example, did you know that Taco Bell's Chicken Gordita with Nacho Cheese only has 270 calories? Order two of those and you've got a 540 calorie meal that won't destroy your day or make you feel like you're "on a diet" when you're out with friends. Compare that to the Taco Bell Fiesta Taco Salad, which clocks in at a surprising 860 calories and you'll see why it's smart to know a few decent options for each fast food chain. Just in case.

A Simple Dumbbell Workout:
http://www.menshealth.com/fitness/dumbbell-exercises-3

This *Men's Health Magazine* article outlines some great, dead simple dumbbell exercises you can do from your home. I don't recommend buying the book they're trying to sell, just memorize a couple of the exercises and incorporate them into a routine of your own design.

Overeaters Anonymous:
http://www.oa.org/

This non-profit group works just like AA or NA, except it exists to help people who can't control their compulsive eating. I've attended a few meetings over the years, but never worked the full recovery program. It's a great group and can be a valuable resource, if you're in the right mindset or if you just need a motivational boost by interacting face-to-fact with some other people who are struggling with their weight and who understand your situation.

www.ingramcontent.com/pod-product-compliance
Lightning Source LLC
Chambersburg PA
CBHW05051529052b

45786CB00007B/2579